Better Sleep Ultimate Guide!

Sleep

Boost Brain Power, Energy, Productivity, And Health With 50 Proven Tips To Stop Insomnia And Fall Asleep Fast!

Mick McPherson

STOP!!! Before you read any further....Would you like to know the secrets of becoming a meditation expert?

If your answer is YES, YES PICK ME you are not alone. Thousands of people are learning the incredible benefits of meditation and how it can help you gain control in your mental and physical life.

If you have been searching for these answers for gaining better understanding about meditation and the secrets to mastering this skill, you have stumbled upon the right place!

Not only will you gain incredible insight in this book, but because I want to make sure to give you as much value as possible, right now you can get full **100% FREE access to a VIP bonus Ebook** on the **Secrets of Becoming A Meditation Expert in 7 Days or Less!**

Just Go Here For Free Instant Access:

www.MeditateMind.com

Legal Notice

Disclaimer Notice

Table Of Contents

Introduction

I want to thank you and congratulate you for purchasing the book, *"Sleep: Better Sleep Ultimate Guide! - Boost Brain Power, Energy, Productivity, And Health With 50 Proven Tips To Stop Insomnia And Fall Asleep Fast!"*

This "Sleep" book contains proven steps and strategies on how to determine if you really have insomnia, implement some easy remedies for it, and help improve the power of your brain, energy, and productivity in the process. If you are having difficulty sleeping, you must not resort to the use of medications right away. There are natural ways of getting the right quantity and quality of sleep. Many of these are already being used by a lot of people out there today. It only takes simple effort on the part of an individual like you to discover what such sleeping problem solutions are.

Of course, you have to look at the right places and access the right informational materials if you don't want to waste your time. You'll discover that there are many tips, techniques, and secrets on how to naturally conquer sleep problems. The number of sources and information could be quite overwhelming. It is for this reason that this book was put together.

Indeed, it is understandable that you want an easy way out of your sleeping problem. This could be the answer to your current need! Use the information presented here in the right way and you'll surely see positive results. Make no mistake about it as this book doesn't guarantee magical or instant results. It will just give you the necessary knowledge, references, and direction in solving your sleeping problem.

You'll be put on the right track when it comes to curing insomnia naturally as well as on establishing and maintaining healthy sleeping habits. The rest will be up to you. Earning the best positive results will require good amounts of effort, dedication, and discipline. However, it will be worth it all in the end.

Thanks again for purchasing this book, I hope you enjoy it!

Chapter 1: Signs And Symptoms Of Sleep Insomnia

Are you having difficulty in sleeping? Most probably, you are wondering if you already have insomnia. While it is really always advisable that you go to a medical professional for an accurate diagnosis, there are things that could be done first. The logic here is that your condition might not be actually chronic or a full blown insomnia but just its "manageable form" that can be remedied at home. Another thing is that the services of such professionals would cost money right away.

There are many instances wherein availing of professional help isn't necessary. An individual could make use of proven ways of overcoming sleep insomnia as discovered by others out there. There are also guides produced and provided by experts on natural cures for sleeping problems.

The first step in conquering sleep insomnia is actually all about determining if you have it or not. The good thing is that there are signs and symptoms that we could use for this matter. There is no need for a medical professional at this point in time. These signs and symptoms could easily be spotted even by an individual like you who has no specialized medical training.

Consider the following:

- *Remain awake for an unusually long period of time before falling asleep*: The normal pattern is for an individual to fall asleep within 15-30minutes of retiring in bed. If it takes you an hour or more to do so, then there is something to be worried about.
- *Waking up continuously after short periods during the entire night*: It involves being easily awakened by slight sounds even if you are already used to such things in the past. This could be explained by the

shallow type of sleep that you are able to achieve. A recent survey revealed some self-diagnosed insomniacs who could wake up and sleep back by as much as 30 times per night.

- **Pattern of deviation from the normal waking hours**: We all know that it is normal for an individual to get a sleeping time of 6 − 8 hours. Of course, you have a normal waking time most especially if you are getting the normal 6-8 hours of sleep. If you keep on observing that you are waking up unusually early for a period of 5 to 10 days, this is something that warrants attention.

- **Unusual tiredness even after sleeping for the entire night**: Sleep is supposed to be our body's mechanism to get recharged and feel ready for activities. However, insomnia could leave you tired, restless, and sleepy even after sleeping through the night. These things are felt throughout the day and you will notice that you are already having a hard time focusing and concentrating on tasks. Clumsiness and forgetfulness are also effects of the "after-sleep tiredness".

- **Feelings of depression and irritability**: During the day, you feel that you are easily upset even by small things that you used to tolerate effectively. This stems from the symptoms of insomnia as mentioned above.

- **Uncomfortable feeling in the stomach accompanied by headaches**: Such symptoms are manifested right when you wake up and increases in intensity as you go through the day.

- **Growing worry or fear about not being able to fall asleep easily**: You are aware that you are not getting enough rest and sleep yet you feel helpless about the situation. The presence of fears about insomnia is most likely an indication that the sleep disorder is actually already there.

Take note of the fact that once a person deviates from the normal patterns of sleeping and resting habits, it could be an indication of insomnia. You are supposed to get 6-8 hours of sleep, wake up feeling refreshed and energetic, and go through the day with a positive aura. If you feel that something is off on your normal habits or resting patterns; go through the list mentioned above. It will provide more affirmation of the presence of your sleeping problem.

Chapter 2: Relaxation Techniques

It is a normal thing to be worried when you are obviously having sleeping problems. Most of us will resort right away to the use of sleeping pills. Indeed, these pills might be effective but this option doesn't really cure the cause of the problem. In the long run, the body could develop an immune reaction to the quantity of sleeping pills that you are taking. This leads to addiction.

It is scientifically proven that a tense body and mind are precursors to sleeping problems. For this reason, the remedy for it could be as simple as performing relaxation exercises. Again, these exercises will take time to learn and get used to. The rewards are there all right. It might not matter that much but when you are already experiencing chronic insomnia; the comfort that it can provide will mean everything.

Relaxation techniques for purposes of sleep problem remediation and improvement of sleep quality will vary greatly. This is something that would depend on the area of expertise of the person being asked. Tips and techniques are found all over the internet. To make things simple for you, only the most effective techniques have been included on this chapter.

A. Mind Relaxation Techniques

1. <u>Thought Filtration</u> – This technique involves the stoppage or removal of thoughts that distract and keep your mind awake. When you find yourself thinking about these types of thoughts, control it and cast it away. Mentally cry out words such as "stop", "don't", or even "away" to clear your mind of these mind distractors.

2. <u>Purpose Reversal</u> – The more that you worry about not being able to fall asleep, the more it will aggravate your insomnia. Instead of doing this, try to aim to be awake as long as possible. The task could actually fool your body into falling asleep.

3. <u>Tension Exhalation</u> – This is a breathing technique that many of us are quite familiar with. Breathe deeply and slowly. Visualize your tension being exhaled out for every cycle of breathing.

4. <u>Float Thought</u> – As the name of the technique implies, you should lie down on your bed and imagine your body to be floating. This is to be done with your eyes closed. Think of your body as a floating feather, an escalator moving in slow motion, or a cloud slowly meeting the ground.

5. <u>Sleep Counting</u> – You probably have seen this on television and in the movies. Yes, it works but you have to visualize the numbers being written by a calligrapher in a very slow but steady motion.

6. <u>Vivid Imagery Generation</u> – You should create pictures of anything that would calm your mind. It can be a beach, a garden with flowers, or a perfectly calm snow covered mountain side. The secret here is to be as attentive as possible even to the tiniest detail. Try to involve as many senses as possible in the process. This is one of the most effective ways to get your mind relaxed in preparation for sleep.

B. Body Relaxation Techniques

1. Massage –This is an effective way to relax tensed and tired muscles. It will become even more effective if done by a professional or when combined with the use of aromatherapy techniques.

2. PMR (Progressive Muscle Relaxation) – Slowly tense your muscle and relax it afterwards. Do this for each muscle group in your body. Best results can be achieved if you will start from your toes and work progressively upwards.

3. Exercise – Light exercise before bedtime releases endorphins within the body. It could induce sleep and make your night rest period really relaxing. Best forms of exercise include yoga and tai-chi.

A relaxed mind and body, when achieved by an individual like you, could make the task of falling asleep almost effortless. Try to use one or two of the techniques mentioned above and see which one would match your actual needs. Now that you have learned how to relax, we shall move on to a very important part of sleep which is dreaming.

Chapter 3: How To Have Lucid Dreams: Basic Facts

Dreaming is a normal thing when you have achieved sleep no matter if it is shallow or deep. Most probably, you have already heard about this thing that they call as LD or lucid dreams. Are you intrigued by it? There is a big chance that all you have at this point in time are speculations about LD. Some say that it is really controlled dreaming. There are a few who are claiming that this is actually how an individual achieves OBE or Out of Body Experience. How about you? What are your ideas about lucid dreams?

Let us examine some basic facts about it in this chapter. To make it simple, lucid dreaming is all about being in a dream and having awareness about it. Are you still confused? To simplify it further, an individual experiencing LD is asleep but he or she is aware of the fact that the things being seen, heard, and felt are all part of a dream. Have you ever dreamed that you are flying and then you realized that nothing about it is true and you will never be physically in danger of falling? The mere fact that you acknowledged it as something that exists in your mind and you had fun in process indicates that you lucidly dreamed.

An expert in this field, Frederick Van Eeden, referred to lucid dreams as "mental clarity". True enough, when an individual is having lucid dreams, every detail is remembered with a surprising level of accuracy and clarity. Generally, the state of lucidity is achieved at the middle of a dream. It happens when an individual suddenly realizes that everything happening around couldn't possibly happen under normal circumstances. This realization could happen even if there are no clues present. Experts in sleep research have found out that 10% of all the lucid dreams that you could ever experience will happen upon going back to REM sleep after you have suddenly been awakened.

There are two levels of lucidity that you can achieve when dreaming. These are as follows:

1. **High Level Lucidity (HLL)** – There is a complete awareness that everything that is happening is all a part of a dream that you are in. You have come to an acknowledgement that no physical harm is possible and that at any moment, you'll wake up.
2. **Low Level Lucidity (LLL)** – This type of lucidity is achieved when you are aware to a limited extent that you are dreaming. Here, you haven't realized that you have the power to alter the scenarios present or that there isn't any risk of getting physically harmed in what you are doing.

Now, why are we talking about lucid dreaming? Are there benefits that we could get from the whole thing? Apparently, the answer here is yes. There are many reasons for us to pay attention on learning how to have lucid dreams. Consider the following:

- **Provides room for safe adventure and fun experiences**: LD enables an individual to experience his or her fantasies in a safe environment. Flying, for example, is one of the most common fantasies of a lot of individuals.
- **Helps in overcoming nightmares**: The realization that the feared elements in a dream can actually help an individual to overcome nightmares. Lucid dreams are used by sleep therapists to help an individual face his fears.
- **Prepares individual for real life scenarios**: This is called as rehearsing. The dream could be as realistic as we could ever expect that it is possible to use it for simulation of feared or expected events. Public speaking, sports performances, and even interviews could be rehearsed through LD.
- **Boosts the brain's creative and problem-solving power**: Current LI (Language International) researchers have found out that language students exposed to LD are more receptive to word associations. Lucid dreamers have

also been seen in another research field as bolder in coming up with works of art.

- **Improves physical health**: Lucid dreaming can promote healing within the body. Healing dreams can actually stimulate the body to focus more on repair of injury, practice of physical functions temporary lost due to injuries, or to simply give an injured individual a positive outlook towards his condition.
- **Acts as a source of transcendent experience**: It helps an individual look into the spiritual aspect of existence. The goal of looking for one's life purpose could actually start in lucid dreams.

Lucid dreaming is not only mysterious for many of us but also promises some very intriguing benefits as shown above. Now, how can you achieve lucid dreams on purpose? Turn to the next chapter to learn about it!

Chapter 4: How To Have Lucid Dreams: Effective Techniques

Yes, lucid dreaming feels almost magical for many of us. This leads them to think that it is a difficult thing to learn. In reality, there are no complicated processes involved in learning how to have lucid dreams. Everybody can learn it. Basically, it is a skill that can be developed and gained through practice. Some of us have this capacity to easily go into lucid dreams. Some of us will experience it only by chance. Can you easily remember what you have dreamed about? If your answer is yes, this is good news as it is a success indicator for those who are planning to train in lucid dreaming.

Even if you don't have that natural talent to go into lucid dreams, you can successfully train for it. Your success will depend upon two very important factors. These include your motivation for the training and the amount of effort that you will put into the whole thing. Through the process of experimentation, observation, and continuous perseverance on training, positive results can be fast tracked.

The following techniques are proven to help individuals like you to have lucid dreams with ease:

TECHNIQUE #1: Recall of Dream Details – There are detailed steps that could be accessed from book EWLD (Exploring the World of Lucid Dreaming). However, the basic idea behind this technique is that you should develop the habit of immediately recording the details of your dreams by note taking. This is done immediately after waking up.

TECHNIQUE #2: Verification of Reality - This is a set of exercise that involves testing elements in your environment to see if there are impossible events that are happening. As an example, you could use your cellphone as a tool to tell time. Look at it and note the time. Look away for a few seconds and see if there will be impossible changes that would happen on the numbers, time, or even text.

TECHNIQUE #3: Identification of "Dream Signs" - This technique has its roots in the EWLD and has been further given attention in other related books. This technique trains you to study your dreams and its detailed elements. Signs that you are dreaming could be easily identified. Examples include a flying house, talking cats, or a never-ending road. You can remind yourself before sleeping that if you see these in your dreams, you'll be reminded that you are in a state of lucidity.

TECHNIQUE #4: The MILD Method – MILD means Mnemonic Induction of Lucid Dreams. On this technique, you will train yourself to remember to do a specific set of action once you have achieved lucidity. You will do this after being awakened from a dream and right before you return to sleep. It consists of three steps:

- Setting up a dream that you want to recall
- Concentrating on your intent to recall everything in the dream you just had
- Voluntary induction to lucidity by thought suggestion and use of dream signs

TECHNIQUE #5: Planned and Timed Napping – There are two approaches on this technique that you can do. First, aim to have lucid dreams during the afternoon. Your chances of success will be higher than when taking morning naps. Another approach is to interject wakefulness periods within your normal periods of sleeping during the night. It works like this:

- Wake up an hour earlier from your normal waking time.
- Stay up for at least 30-60 minutes while doing technique 1, 2, 3, and 4.
- Resume sleeping.

The success that you'll get from these techniques will vary

depending on your dedication to attaining gradual results and on the consistency of your training. Now that you have learned techniques in achieving lucid dreams, it is time for you to move on to sleep meditations. The next chapter will give you all the pertinent sets of information about it.

Chapter 5: Sleep Meditations

If you have been through one of those sleepless nights, you'll definitely agree that putting the mind at rest in order to fall asleep is more difficult to do than what you may have originally thought. The second chapter of this book taught you some mind and body relaxation techniques. However, attaining a relaxed mind and body is just the start of getting the quality and quantity of sleep that is labeled as ideal. Our ability to control thoughts at will plays a more significant role in the attainment of such a goal.

Meditation is one of the best ways around the dilemma being mentioned above. You'll discover that as the night goes deeper and you are still awake, frustration levels increase and anxiety sets in. This is what disturbs the flow of thoughts that you have. As you can see, thought processes that have been slowed down through conscious efforts would pave the way to the initiation of a truly restful sleep.

The effectiveness of meditation in helping us sleep and overcome insomnia would depend on many factors. One is about the amount of practice that you are willing to do. Most of the time, you have to practice meditation techniques many times throughout the day before you can get any good progress during the night. Sleeping pattern is another factor here. There are people who are used to staying up 4 hours or more before feeling relaxed and ready to sleep. Some are able to fall asleep just after a few minutes of lying down in bed.

The biggest factor here, however, is the kind of meditation that would be chosen. There are different types of meditation that you could choose from. The types that promote mental alertness should be avoided. Such meditation types include those that are taught in yoga, Zen, and tai-chi. By doing these meditation types 15 minutes before going to bed; you will reduce your chances of immediately falling asleep.

The most recommended type is under the broad category called as "mindful-meditation". It basically slows down the flow of thoughts coming into your mind. It also gives you the power to put the pace of your thoughts on the right track in case it wanders off. We all have this thing called as "inner chatter" in our minds and if this can be controlled (slowed down or calmed down); we can achieve that greater level of relaxation. After this, you can proceed to specific types of meditation that could match your actual needs.

Under the "mindful-meditation" category, three very effective techniques could be used for the attainment of high quality sleep. You can try out any of the following:

1. *Mindful Breathing Technique*–The process is quite easy as you will just pay attention to the pattern of your natural breathing. By doing this, you actually take your mind off thoughts that could disrupt the process of falling asleep. This is most effective if used together with music and guided visual imagery.

2. *Body Scan Technique* – This is very similar to the PMR (Progressive Muscle Relaxation) method mentioned on the 2nd chapter of this book. Start out by using technique #1 and then turn your attention to your toes. Visualize and feel it getting heavy and sinking into the bed. Move up and do the whole process all over again on your lower leg. Proceed upwards until you have "scanned" all of your body.

3. *Combination Style Technique*: As the name suggests, you can choose parts of different meditation and relaxation techniques here. Just remember to avoid those that add up to the alertness level of your mind and body. You can refer to chapter 2 of this book for a complete list of those techniques that can be combined.

Before you try any of the techniques mentioned above, it is necessary that you set realistic expectations about the results that can be obtained. If you haven't tried meditation yet, practice it. The help of a professional sleep therapist will definitely help, but it is not a requirement.

Chapter 6: Exercises To Help Improve Sleep Quality

The link between exercise and sleep quality has been one of the most researched topics for the past few years. It is very obvious that the process of energy usage required in heavy physical activities such as in exercises could explain its link to sleep. Tiredness leads to your body's need to rest and sleep. This is something that can be done without much of an effort. However, if there are already sleeping pattern disruptions or insomnia has already manifested itself, the use of exercise becomes magnified.

So what are the things that researchers have found out about exercise and sleep? The following are just some of their most significant findings:

- Exercise time that reaches the mark of 150 minutes per week leads to better feeling and significant amounts of sleep among individuals.
- Among the elderly, the effects of an exercise program will not show immediate effects in the sleep patterns. The effects will come gradually and will tend to last for long periods of time.
- The inclusion of exercises to routine activities produces more positive results in terms of sleep quality and duration.
- Young individuals who get engaged in heavy physical activities such as those involved in sport fall asleep faster than their less active peers.
- Exercising in the afternoon results to a more restful sleep in the evening.
- A period of adjustment for the body must be allocated if a new physical activity routine is to be added to the existing daily activities.

Generally, any activity or exercise that uses up the body's store of energy will do if you are looking for a way to prepare for sleeping disorder remediation. You can do aerobics, jogging, cycling, or any other heavy physical activity during the day. The logic here is simple: drain away your energy stores and the body will respond naturally to replenish it through hunger, thirst, and of course sleep. Just remember that there are rules which you should follow when exercising for the purpose of falling asleep or improving sleep quality. These are as follows:

> **Rule #1**: Boost up aerobic exercise time by adding 20 to 30 minutes of activity.

> **Rule #2:** Do your exercises before having dinner.

> **Rule #3**: Exercise should be intense but balanced in a way that the body will not become overworked.

> **Rule #4:** Any daily routine activity could be turned into an exercise by increasing the time allocated for it. For example, if you are walking your dog daily for 10 minutes daily, extend it to 20 minutes by taking a longer route.

The physical activities that are mentioned above are supposed to be done 6 hours before bedtime. It is recommended that when you are already in bed, only stretching exercises should be done. Some examples of these exercises include the following:

- *"Swan at Rest"*–With a pillow in front of you, sit down with your right leg brought towards the inner thigh and the left leg extended straight towards the back. Hinge your body forward and let your head touch the pillow. Hold this for 8-10 seconds. Reverse position of legs and repeat the steps above.
- *"Baby in Bed"* – Do this by lying flat on the bed. Bring your knees up to the chest and hold the inner side of your feet. Move your knees to the left side and then to right. Keep knees and feet flexed on each side for 10 seconds.
- *"Raised Bridge"* – Lie flat on your back; bend your knees with your feet on the bed or floor. Your hands should be on your sides with palms facing down. Use your shoulders as

the anchor point. Gently raise your hips so that it forms a diagonal line with the shoulders. Hold this for 10 seconds.

- *"Lateral Benders"* – Sit cross-legged on your bed. Raise both of your hands above the head. Lower left hands, palms facing down, to the bed. With your right hand still extended above your head, lean towards the left side. Hold this position for 10 seconds. Reverse hand positions repeat the process.
- *"Bent Doll Carry"* – Stand up straight with both feet slightly apart. Place left hand on right elbow and right hand on left elbow. Bend your hips and let the upper body hang down naturally (like a doll being carried by the waist). Hold this position for 10 seconds.

With these exercises completed, your body should be ready to get its much-needed preparation for rest and sleep. We will now proceed to an important skill that you should learn: calming the mind. Chapter 7 contains all the information you need about this matter.

Chapter 7: How To Calm Your Mind

One of the possible reasons why you are having this difficulty on falling asleep is that because you have an overactive mind. Most probably, you have experienced lying in bed and trying to fall asleep while constant streams of thoughts are coming. Thoughts about the bills, upcoming paperwork deadlines, your kid's problems at school, the disturbing news you just saw on TV and all other things are keeping you awake.

Is it possible to "shut the brain" before bedtime? By this, we mean stopping the flow of thoughts that disturb the current level of relaxation that you have. Calming the mind is apparently easier said than done. There are mind calming techniques that can be learned but if these are done incorrectly, it would just result to a greater state of wakefulness.

The following techniques are proven to work both for those who have an "overactive" and "average-paced" mind:

- **Distraction**: To overcome thoughts that trigger excitement and wakefulness, distract your mind with things that can bore it. Examples include:
    - ✓ Imagine a flock of sheep and try to count each one slowly.
    - ✓ Go through the letters of the alphabet and pick an example for each.
    - ✓ Visualize a long trip and everything that you will see while on it.
    - ✓ Go through your fantasies (like going to the moon, spending a million dollars, etc.). The logic here is that you will trick your mind into not entertaining thoughts about problems for the day.
- **Routine**: Creating and following a pre-sleep routine has been proven to effectively calm the mind in preparation for sleep. This routine is a way of the mind on winding down.

The body recognizes activities that are meant for day or night. A pre-sleep routine basically signals the start of the night activities which includes rest and sleep. When your mind and body has been "tuned" down, falling asleep becomes an easy thing to do. It is ideal that you allocate 30 minutes for pre-sleep routine before you actually try to sleep. Examples of these routines include:

- ✓ Reading a book (under a genre that won't excite you.)
- ✓ Listening to music (Relaxing type)
- ✓ Drinking a glass of warm milk.
- ✓ Light stretching routines.
- ✓ Journal or diary writing.

- ***Environment Optimization***: The mind responds well to the types of stimuli that the environment will feed it. This is where you can have complete control. Prepare your bedroom for sleeping by creating a relaxing ambiance. Tone down the lighting level, make sure that it is properly ventilated and cool, quiet, and if possible, has an aromatic odor from fragrance candles lit earlier and then put out.

These are not the only techniques that can help you attain a calm mind. As you go on exploring the causes of your sleeping problems, you will come across many possible solutions. Most of the time, those things will work only for your case. List down what works for you and what should be avoided. In general, getting the mind calmed should be easy if those techniques mentioned above and those that you will discover would be applied.

Chapter 8: Intimacy And Sleep Quality

Most probably, you've heard about this very controversial issue about the link between intimacy and sleep quality. There are many people who value close relationships and they claim that it is just natural for us to share a bed with a partner or spouse. Doing so will lead to peace of mind, feeling of being loved, and of course restful nights of sleep. However, there are researches that revealed the opposite thing. According to some recent findings by sleep researchers, intimacy and the resulting decision to share beds with our loved ones could affect the quality of sleep that we are getting.

With these two contradicting ideas around, we are bound to be confused on what to believe. Should you share a bed with your partner? Will it be better if you and your partner sleep apart? These questions have suddenly become hard to answer now. At the modern era that we are in, it is hard to deny that people who have spouses or intimate partners are finding more reasons to sleep away from each other.

Take for example the difference in work scenarios and personal habits when sleeping. If you are an early bird and your partner is a late-night owl, both of you will have an impact on each other's sleep pattern. If it is your habit to sleep early and your partner likes to stay up and watch late night TV shows, this could end up in you not getting enough sleep.

Your sleeping conditions such as snoring, waking up frequently due to sleeping disorders, and even sleepwalking could lead to a low quality of sleep for your partner. You should remember that disruptions in sleep have negative health effects such as diabetes, obesity, heart and lung problems, and unstable emotional conditions. Such things have a big role in developing troubled relationships between couples.

On the other side of the issue, there are experts who disagree on the whole idea of couples totally separating their bedrooms. The bed that is shared is a symbol of closeness, of sharing, and commitment to the relationship. Of course, there are also studies that discovered that intimacy with a partner relaxes the mind and provides emotional calmness Of course, logically, sexual activities that happen before sleeping spends considerable amounts of energy on both sides, this could be good for those who want to fall asleep right away.

Even with the explanations of the good side of sharing a bed and providing a chance for intimacy, many couples these days still find it easy to choose this so-called "bed divorce". For many of them, this is the only way that they can really improve their sleep quality.

If you are also planning on doing or suggesting this to your partner, it is good to look into some alternative solutions. One of these is about exploring the real cause of the poor quality sleep that both of you are getting. Have you looked into the real cause of your sleep disorder? It could be your lifestyle, your diet, and vices that are causing your insomnia. Have you thought about the environment of your bedroom? Lights must have been set too bright. There could be sources of distraction in the room such as the presence of a TV, a noisy air conditioning unit, or even a heater that is not producing the right temperature.

It is true that your partner's sleep patterns, habits, and behavior could affect the quality of your sleep. However, this thing called sleep divorce is not the only solution here. Both of you must sit down and talk things out. There are always ways on which differences on sleep patterns and habits between couples could be settled. After all, it is your partner with whom you will share that bed for the rest of your life as a couple. Make it work and see your sleep quality improve in the long run.

Chapter 9: 50 Tips To Stop Insomnia

Insomnia can ruin your health and relationships with others. Prevention and cure methods are always being explored continuously by experts. From time to time, we will hear about new innovations about insomnia solutions. These are added to those things that the public already knows. If you are looking for a simple compilation of tips that can be used to stop insomnia, this chapter has it all for you.

The following are 50 of the most effective tips on preventing, stopping, and curing insomnia:

1. Try doing some relaxation routines before you go to bed. It could be about reading some books or taking a short stroll down your neighborhood.
2. Don't bring paperwork to the bed. If possible, your work table shouldn't be in the bedroom.
3. Remove the television from your bedroom. It will just tempt you to stay up late.
4. Wear a headset or earplugs if there are noises that penetrate through your room.
5. Decorate or set up your room in the same manner as those places that you find relaxing.
6. Don't take medicines that have stimulants added in as ingredients.
7. See to it that your home HVAC or ventilation unit is giving you the right temperature.
8. The number of blankets on your bed should be limited.
9. Explore a sleeping position that always makes falling asleep easy for you. Stick to it.
10. Choose a mattress that effectively supports the body according to weight distribution. A sagging mattress should be avoided.
11. Pick a bed that will provide enough space for you and your partner. Remember sleeping positions could change while you are sleeping.
12. Wear something comfortable. Some people find sleeping naked beneficial to their sleep quality.

13. Try to determine if you will sleep better with or without pillows.
14. If you are a "lights on" sleeper, make sure that your lampshade or bedroom lights have a "soft lights" setting.
15. If you prefer to sleep in the dark, see to it that your curtains are made up of heavy materials.
16. Wake up and go to bed at the same time per day. This way, the body can get used to the routine very easily.
17. Rise up immediately when you wake up. It gives your body a message that the bed is meant to be for sleep purposes only.
18. Long naps in the late afternoon should be avoided. Power naps (15 minutes maximum) could be taken but not within 6 hours before bedtime.
19. Exercises that require fast consumption of energy (aerobics) should be done within the day.
20. Cut the booze and cigarettes before bedtime. If possible, abstain from these things at least 2-3 hours before going to bed.
21. Instead of drinking caffeinated drinks during dinner, go for water.
22. When watching TV, avoid those shows that excite or stress up the mind.
23. Read books that bore you when you're already in bed.
24. Arguments with other people should be avoided.
25. Pick a sleeping schedule wherein there is a guarantee that no one would bother or disturb you.
26. Salty food items should be avoided. If you cannot avoid it, match your dinner with plenty of water. However, this can lead to frequent bathroom runs throughout the night.
27. A light pre-bedtime snack consisting of milk, cheese, and nuts (provided you are not allergic to any of these items) will be good for you.
28. Calcium supplements could be taken after meal to improve sleep quality.
29. Herb-based teas provide a relaxing effect on the body. Take it if you don't want milk before bedtime.
30. Mix a bit of brewer's yeast and molasses (1 teaspoon each) into a glass of warm milk you will drink before going to bed.
31. Remove clutter from your nightstand. It helps to relax your mind in preparation for sleep.

32. Don't focus too much on the thought that you need to fall asleep.
33. Keep a log or list of your worries and then forget everything about it when you go to bed. Deal with those things in the morning.
34. Drink a glass of warm water mixed with a teaspoon of honey or the "traditional bedtime mix" consisting of equal amounts of honey and cider vinegar mixed with warm water.
35. Allow your partner to point out which sleeping position you tend to sleep with fewer disruptions (snoring, frequent waking up, etc.) and try to stick to it when you are trying to sleep.
36. Aim for realistic number of sleeping hours (4-6 for adults).
37. Don't reflect on the day's events when you are already lying down in bed.
38. Explore if "bed divorce" will work for you and your spouse or partner. If not; just get a bigger bed.
39. Set your bedroom thermostat at 62 degrees Fahrenheit.
40. Take a quick warm shower before bedtime.
41. Maintain a correct level of humidity in your bedroom. It is good to invest in a humidifier device that can be incorporated into your existing HVAC system.
42. Footbaths and massages will help calm your body.
43. Perform a bit of meditation before retiring to bed.
44. Listen to soft music while thinking about calming ideas or sceneries.
45. Have your partner tell you a story that doesn't arouse your interest much.
46. Focus your attention on breathing instead of on your thoughts.
47. Counting is one of the most common tips for one to fall asleep. Yes, it is still effective for that purpose today. Instead of the usual flock of sheep, get creative with other things.
48. Don't go to bed when you haven't yet resolved arguments with your spouse or partner yet. A peaceful state of emotion has been connected by research to better quality of sleep.
49. Don't put your cell phones and other gadgets near your body when sleeping. There are researches that link the radiation emitted by these devices to the brain waves that are needed for a peaceful type of sleep.

50. Have that commitment and determination to stick to a healthy diet and an active lifestyle.

Chapter 10: The Affects Of Diet And Your Sleep

The last part of this book will cover the issue about the effect of diet on sleep. While it might seem obvious that these two are connected, it still matters that you know the specifics of the issue. It will allow you to make some necessary changes on the way that you eat so that insomnia will never set in and you'll always enjoy good quality of sleep each night.

Let us get started on the amount of food that we consume before bedtime. Too much or too little of it will have an effect on our sleep quality. Eat too much and you will make your body work excessively on the process of digestion. Hormones that are meant to put your body and brain to sleep will have a delayed release. Eat too little and your body will allow its natural mechanism of hunger and thirst to wake you up within your sleeping hours.

There are substances that are added to our food that can also disrupt or affect sleep quality. Take for example caffeine which is a very popular additive in drinks and even in energy bars. It is a type of stimulant which will naturally keep the body and brain active if taken an hour or two before bedtime. Alcohol is another "sleep killer". While it is a depressant which lowers brain activity, it could lead to low quality sleep with many interruptions throughout the night.

Some people have this idea of "flushing" out those sleep-quality reducing substances. They think that by drinking a lot of water before bedtime, they are doing something wise. This is not a good idea as it will only increase the possibility of having this need to get up frequently just to pee.

Actually, there are some diet related tips that you can follow if you want to have restful sleep every night. These are as follows:

- Don't skip meals during the day and then try to compensate for it by eating a heavy meal at night. Overeating, as mentioned above, will keep your digestive system extra active all night. This leads to difficulty in falling asleep or frequently disturbed sleep during the night.
- Carbs should not be ruled out when you are preparing dinner. Carbohydrates are needed for the production of tryptophan which is a "sleep inducing hormone".
- Your diet should not be highlighted with extreme amounts of nutrients. It means that these nutrients should not go beyond or below the standard amounts. The same goes for the amount of calories you are getting on a daily basis.
- Go light on processed foods. Such food items contain substances that are precursors to health conditions such as diabetes, hypertension, and obesity.
- Aim for a dinner menu with food items rich in B-vitamins, calcium, zinc, copper, and iron. These are vitamins and minerals that are proven to help relax the mind and lead to good quality of sleep.
- Slowly introduce the use of herbs into your diet. This is of course if you cannot directly go for a full herbal way of life. As an example, instead of drinking coffee after a meal, try chamomile tea.
- Eating more frequently in small amounts is good. You can keep your weight in check and ensure that obesity will never set in. Obesity is one of the leading causes of sleep problems among individuals today.

It is not difficult at all to see the link between diet and our sleep. If you want to avoid insomnia and to always enjoy the right quality of sleep, the best thing to do is to maintain a healthy diet. Remember, you must eat right in order to sleep right.

Conclusion

Thank you again for purchasing this book on *"Sleep: Better Sleep Ultimate Guide! - Boost Brain Power, Energy, Productivity, And Health With 50 Proven Tips To Stop Insomnia And Fall Asleep Fast!"*

I am extremely excited to pass this information along to you, and I am so happy that you now have read and can hopefully implement these strategies going forward.

I hope this book was able to help you understand the process of fighting and preventing insomnia and how to achieve restful nights of sleep.

The next step is to get started using this information and to hopefully live an energetic, productive, and inspiration-driven life!

Please don't be someone who just reads this information and doesn't apply it, the strategies in this book will only benefit you if you use them!

If you know of anyone else that could benefit from the information presented here please inform them of this book.

Finally, if you enjoyed this book and feel it has added value to your life in any way, please take the time to share your thoughts and post a review on Amazon. It'd be greatly appreciated!

Thank you and good luck!

Preview Of:

Ultimate NLP Techniques Guide!

<u>NLP Techniques</u>

Neuro Linguistic Programming And Neuroplasticity Strategies To Overcome Fear, Increase Self Esteem, Self Confidence, Motivation, And Inner Peace!

Introduction

I want to thank you and congratulate you for purchasing the book, "NLP Techniques: Ultimate NLP Techniques Guide! - Neuro Linguistic Programming And Neuroplasticity Strategies To Overcome Fear, Increase Self Esteem, Self Confidence, Motivation, And Inner Peace!"

This book contains proven steps and strategies on how to be able to use different NLP techniques and strategies in order to help you improve your thoughts, gain new skills, and become more aware of your behavior patterns so that you can improve or change them to have a better method of doing your activities. At the same time, this book will also help you remove bad habits and help you gain inner peace.

This book is made for people who want to discover how far they can go and how they are going to take control of their life. NLP would help you become aware that you can be limitless as long as your mind is capable of stretching itself in order for you to realize your full potential. Now, you are going to be the person that you want to be by having a mind that will constantly work to improve you.

Thanks again for purchasing this book. I hope you enjoy it!

Chapter 1: Basics Of NLP And Neuro Linguistic Programming

Imagine this scenario: There is a screen in front of you which shows that you are walking barefoot in a garden and you can feel the freshly-cut grass underneath your feet. You see that there is a snake lying on the grass. At the right side of the screen is a button, which is labeled "Transmogrify." Press that button. When you look back at the screen, you will see that the snake has turned into a rope.

What you just did is a part of neuro linguistic programming, or NLP. This technique is one of the most popular methods in psychology, which aims to allow a person to be in control of his thoughts, actions, and bodily functions simply by changing the way his mind works.

Why People Like the Idea

The entire concept of NLP has been embraced by psychologists, counselors, doctors, and teachers because it is extremely practical. By having a technique that can actually help people help themselves, you can probably imagine how it can make people save up time and money just for them to find a fix with their problems.

NLP has been introduced as a means to "program" one's mindset and behavior through linguistic and behavioral patterns. People also believe that it is possible for them to also predict patterns and calculate consequences simply by being able to manipulate one's mind through a series of actions. Why is it called as such? Neuro refers to the manner that the mind and body interacts. Linguistic refers to the way that a person can be influenced through certain language patterns, and programming refers to the patterns of behavior and thinking (or programs) that people prefer to use to put order in their daily lives.

So what does this say about human behavior? That means that it is possible for people to actually change the way they see the world around them by changing the way they think and behave. It means that it is possible for people to get over their fears, make sure that they are motivated, get over stress and anxiety, simply by changing the way they react towards certain stimulus.

Richard Bandler, one of the proponents of NLP, thinks that anyone can do NLP. It doesn't require for one to have studied behavioral psychology or have a degree in logic and mathematics to actually study it. For that reason, there are hundreds of books out there that provide certain NLP exercises that the most ordinary people can do to make sure that they can help themselves rewire their mind, with them holding the control. While it is not designed to replace physicians and behavioral experts, it provides that general idea that when people need help getting over thoughts and change their behavior, they can have a manual to do that that they can afford.

What Can NLP Do?

NLP is essentially a set of methods, insights, and skills that allows you to take charge of what you feel and think which is very essential to have when you want to be the one running your own life. Being skilled in this technique allows you to do the following:

1. Think more clearly and be able to see situations as they really

are.

2. Communicate your thoughts more effectively.

3. Have control of your emotions, moods, behavior, impulses, and thoughts.

4. Be able to acquire and develop more skills and become efficient in doing tasks.

Now that you know what this practice is trying to achieve, you will learn more about how NLP works in the next chapter.

Thanks for Previewing My Exciting Book Entitled:

"NLP Techniques: Ultimate NLP Techniques Guide! Neuro Linguistic Programming And Neuroplasticity Strategies To Overcome Fear, Increase Self Esteem, Self Confidence, Motivation, And Inner Peace!"

To purchase this book, simply go to the Amazon Kindle store and simply search:

"NLP TECHNIQUES"

Then just scroll down until you see my book. You will know it is mine because you will see my name "Mick McPherson" underneath the title.

Alternatively, you can visit my author page on Amazon to see this book and other work I have done. Thanks so much, and please don't forget your free bonuses

DON'T LEAVE YET! - CHECK OUT YOUR FREE BONUSES BELOW!

Free Bonus Offer: Get Free Access To The www.MeditateMind.com VIP Newsletter!

Once you enter your email address you will immediately get free access to this awesome newsletter!

But wait, right now if you join now for free you will also get free access the "Secrets of Becoming A Meditation Expert – In 7 Days!" free Ebook!

To claim both your FREE VIP NEWSLETTER MEMBERSHIP and your FREE BONUS Ebook on the SECRETS OF BECOMING A MEDITATION EXPERT IN 7 DAYS!

Just Go To:

www.MeditateMind.com